Juicing

I0422008

111 Delicious Juicing Recipes For Weight Loss, Increasing Metabolism, And To Detox Your Body Naturally To Increase Overall Health, Natural Beauty, And Energy!

Chris Smith

STOP!!! Before you read any further....Would you like to know the Secrets of Body Transformation?

If your answer is yes, then you are not alone. Thousands of people are looking for the secret to rapidly burn body fat, keep the weight off, become healthier, and truly transform their body and life for good.

If you have been searching for these answers without much luck, you are in the right place!

Not only will you gain incredible insight in this book, but because I want to make sure to give you as much value as possible, right now for a limited time you can get full **100% FREE access to a VIP bonus EBook** entitled **THE 7 KEYS TO BODY TRANSFORMATION!**

Just Go Here For Free Instant Access:

www.liveFitVIP.com

Legal Notice

Disclaimer Notice

Table Of Contents

Introduction

I want to thank you and congratulate you for purchasing the book, "Juicing - Delicious Juicing Recipes For Weight Loss, Increasing Metabolism, And To Detox Your Body Naturally To Increase Overall Health, Natural Beauty, And Energy!"

This "Juicing" e-book contains proven steps and strategies on how to make delicious and nutritious juice.

Fresh vegetable and fruit juice is much healthier than regular soda that is full of sugar and artificial ingredients. Most commercially produced juice drinks are actually mislabeled. Manufacturers claim that they are "freshly squeezed" when in fact, the juices have been extracted and then stored for months and even years. They just treat the mixture with color and flavoring prior to packing. They lack nutrients in truly freshly squeezed juice so making your own juice is essential if you wish to get the full benefits.

The juicing process removes the insoluble fiber from the fruits and vegetables. Fiber has its own benefits but it can also slow down the absorption of nutrients in the body. Juices are beneficial for people who cannot consume whole fruits. Children are also more comfortable drinking juice than eating vegetables. If there is a particular vegetable that you do not enjoy, you can juice it and add other sweet fruits to mask the flavor.

Drinking fresh juice can help you adapt a healthier lifestyle. For those who are not used to consuming fresh fruits and vegetables, juicing is a creative and delicious way to increase your vegetable consumption. This book contains many juicing recipes that provide many health benefits. There are also some tips and trick that can help you get started.

Thanks again for purchasing this book, I hope you enjoy it!

Chapter 1: Benefits Of Juicing

People who are not a fan of whole produce can benefit from juicing vegetables and fruits.It is also great to add to your detoxification and weight loss program.

A convenient way to meet nutritional requirements

The recommended consumption for fruits and vegetables is 5-7 servings in a day. Some people may not be able to consume a lot of produce if they simply eat whole foods. Juice is easier to consume that whole vegetables and fruits.

Incredibly healthy

Juice from whole produce contains more vitamins and nutrients than other beverages. Fruits and vegetables are rich in antioxidants that can protect the body from free radicals. It can even replace your regular energy drinks. Fresh juice is easily absorbed by the body so it provides instant nourishment when you need it.

Make your own special blend

You can be creative in making your own juice. Start by using ingredients that you are familiar with. You can start with a simple recipe, and then gradually add more ingredients. Making your own juice also allows you to control the additives that you mix. You can completely remove sugar for a healthier drink or you can also use natural sweeteners like honey and maple syrup to make it more palatable.

What should you expect?

Once you start consuming high quality foods like fresh fruits and vegetables, your body will start to get rid of inferior materials from processed foods to make room for healthier materials. Your body might need to adjust to the changes. The most common effect of this regeneration process is lethargy or decrease in energy. This happens when the body is trying to recuperate and get rid of the toxins. Be persistent and patient because this will only last for about 3-5 days.

Chapter 2: List Of What You Will Need To Get Started With Juicing

Juicing fruits and vegetables is a great way to improve your health. Many diet experts say that consuming fresh juice for a few days can help your body eliminate toxins from processed foods.

Juicing is relatively easy to do and most people already have the necessary equipment in their house.

A high power juicer

The main equipment that you need is a high-power juicer that can churn fruits and vegetables. Look for one that runs on at least 800 watts of power. This amount of power can separate juice from the pulp of the fruits and vegetables. Fortunately, there are a lot of juicers to choose from depending on your budget. It is also good a great advantage if the juicer is easy to disassemble and clean.

Refrigerator/Freezer

You can make a large batch of juice and keep it in your refrigerator until ready to drink. This can preserve the nutrients in the juice. Having a ready supply of juice in your refrigerator can be convenient. You can also use the refrigerator to store whole fruits and vegetables until you are ready to juice it.

Lots and lots of fruits and vegetables

You need fruits and vegetables to create your juice. Make a list of the ingredients that you need and try to buy in bulk to help you save money. Make sure to purchase sweet fruits like apple, banana and mango since these are regularly added to the recipes.

Chapter 3: Things That You Need To Know Before You Make 111 Delicious Juice Recipes

Here are some of the things that you have to keep in mind before your start juicing:

When to drink your juice

The best time to drink fresh juice is on an empty stomach or at least 30 minutes before eating. This is the time where your stomach readily absorbs anything that you eat.

Do not worry about consuming citrus fruits in the morning because it actually has alkalizing effect on the body. Your stomach can also adapt to drinking large amount of juice.

As a general rule, it is best to drink fruit juices during the first half of the day to control your appetite and to keep you energized. Drink juices that are not too sweet like green juice for the later part of the day.

What to juice

People who are new to juicing should start with fruits and vegetables that they like. This can help you adjust to the taste and texture of the juice. Start with common produce that is easily digested like apples, carrots and watermelons.

Remember that the greener the vegetable, the healthier and less palatable it is. Once you are ready for green juice, you may need to add natural sweetener like honey or sweet fruits like banana and apple.

Rotate fruits and vegetables

The body needs adequate amount of nutrients, vitamins, enzymes and amino acid. Eating and drinking a variety of fruits and vegetables ensure that you are getting all the nutrients that you need. Even if you indulge in your favorite recipe, make sure that you still consume other vegetables and fruits.

How safe is that juice?

- The sugar

Fruits are rich in natural sugar that can replace refined sweeteners. Fruit sugar is also low glycemic which means that it does not cause blood sugar fluctuations. You can also dilute the juice with water.

- The pesticides

Commercially grown fruits and vegetables are sprayed with pesticides and chemicals. You can soak the vegetables in a mixture of salt and apple cider vinegar. Leave it for 10 minutes until you notice that the solution starts to smell different. Rinse the vegetables and use it as you wish. You can also opt for organically grown vegetables and fruits.

- The wax

Fruits like apples naturally produce a thin coat of wax that protects the skin of the fruit. In most fruits, nutrients are concentrated under the skin. You can simply peel the skin before eating or juicing it.

Listen to your body

Juicing should be a pleasant experience. Make sure that the taste is pleasant enough to consume. Make sure that you listen to your body. If you feel nauseated or queasy, you may have consumed something that does not agree with your stomach. Drink as much juice as you want as long as you are comfortable with it. You will know once you have consumed enough juice because you might feel 'forced' to drink it. Knowing what to expect can help you understand and prepare for the changes that may affect your body.

Drink the juice you prepared right away

It can take only about 15 minutes to prepare the juice. Remember that once the juice is exposed to air, it loses its nutrients rapidly so make sure that you consume it immediately. Juice that has been exposed to oxidation is no longer safe to drink. You know that it has oxidized if it turns brown. Make sure that you store the juice in an airtight container if you want to serve it later. Make sure to fill the container to the brim so that there will be no space for oxygen.

Clean your juicer properly

One of the factors that you have to consider when choosing a juicer is that it must be easy to assemble and clean. Also, make it a habit to clean your juicer after every use to avoid contamination and bacteria buildup.

To clean, dismantle the juicer and rinse under running water. Use a small brush to remove stuck pieces. You can also clean the inside using a mild solution.

Chapter 4: Juicing Recipes For Weight Loss

1. Tomato and cucumber juice

Ingredients:

1 celery stalk

2 cups tomatoes

½ tsp salt

4 drops stevia

2 cups cucumber, diced

¼ tsp cayenne pepper

Procedure:

Process the ingredients in a juicer.

2. Watercress & carrots

Ingredients:

2 diced tomatoes

Salt and pepper

1 cup watercress

3 carrots

½ cup cilantro

½ cup spinach

Procedure:

Chop the ingredients. Place in a juicer and process.

3. Celery & Beet juice

Ingredients:

1 small beet

5 celery stalks

½ cup cilantro

1 tsp honey

Procedure:

Combine ingredients in a juicer.

4. Spinach & Apple

Ingredients:

2 tbsp lemon juice

½ cup lettuce leaves

3 apples

1 cup spinach

Procedure:

Chop the ingredients. Process it in the juicer.

5. Grapefruit Pepper Juice

Ingredients:

1 grapefruit

7 drop honey

1 yellow pepper

1 kiwi fruit

1 inch ginger, grated

Procedure:

Process it in a juicer then serve.

6. Watermelon Lemon Juice

Ingredients:

1 tsp mint leaves

1 cup watermelon

Juice of 1 lemon

Procedure:

Combine ingredients in a juicer and process.

7. Lychee & Pomegranate Juice

Ingredients:

1 cup lychee

½ cup pomegranate

1 tsp vanilla

Procedure:

Place ingredients in a juicer. Process it then pour in a glass.

8. Refreshing Apple Juice

Ingredients:

3 apples

1 celery stick

1 cup lettuce

1 cup spinach

Procedure:

Chop then place it in the juicer. Pour in a glass and add ice if desired.

9. Vegetable delight

Ingredients:

2 oranges

2 carrots

2 large broccolis

1 celery stick

Procedure:

Juice the oranges first and pour in a glass. Blend the remaining ingredients and mix.

10. Green Juice
Ingredients:

2 carrots

½ cup spinach

1 cucumber

1 celery stick

1 cup kale

Procedure:

Juice ingredients and pour in a glass.

11. Beets and treats
Ingredients:

1 orange

2 cabbage leaf

1 cup spinach

Half lemon

1 beet root

Procedure:

Juice the ingredients and serve cold.

12. Ginger Apple Juice

Ingredients:

2 medium apples

Half lemon

1 inch ginger

1 tbsp honey

Procedure:

Juice the ingredients and pour in a glass.

13. Kale Juice

Ingredients:

5 handful kale

2 apples

1 tbsp honey

2 cups spinach

Procedure:

Juice the fruits and vegetables. Add the honey later for taste.

14. Green Weight Loss Juice

Ingredients:

1 cucumber

6 kale leaves

2 apples

Half lemon

1 cucumber

Procedure:

Juice the ingredients and serve.

15. Skinny Cocktail

Ingredients:

1 cup parsley

2 celery stalks

1 apple

2 oranges

5 kale leaves

Procedure:

Juice the ingredients and pour in a glass.

16. Green Lemonade

Ingredients:

2 apples

4 kale leaves

2 cups spinach

1 cucumber

Procedure:

Process the ingredients in a juicer. Stir then serve.

17. Sunset Blend

Ingredients:

Sweet potato

2 apples

1 beet root

1 orange

Procedure:

Place in a juicer and process.

18. Turmeric Sunrise

Ingredients:

2 apples

Juice of 2 lemons

2 pears

2 carrots

Procedure:

Juice the ingredients.

19. Radiant Red

Ingredients:

2 apples

4 carrots

1 cup dandelion greens

2 kale leaves

1 beet root

1 inch ginger root

1 orange

Procedure:

Process the ingredients in a juicer.

20.   Workout Juice

Ingredients:

1 cup dandelion green

3 kale leaf

2 medium apples

Half cucumber

Juice from half lemon

Procedure:

Juice the fruits and vegetables. Add the lemon juice.

21. Calcium Rich Juice

Ingredients:

3 carrots

1 cup collard greens

1 pepper

1 cup cilantro

1 apple

Procedure:

Process ingredients and serve.

22. Tropical Green Juice

Ingredients:

1 inch ginger root

1 mango

1 cup pineapple

4 kale leaves

Procedure:

Process the ingredients in a juicer.

23. Green Aid
Ingredients:

4 apples

2 kale leaves

3 celery stalks

1 cup pineapple

Procedure:

Juice the ingredients.

24. Fresh Salsa
Ingredients:

1 tsp cayenne pepper

1 garlic clove

1 onion

1 cup tomato

1 medium pepper

Procedure:

Process the ingredients in a juicer.

25. Green and Red Breakfast

Ingredients:

2 apples

1 cucumber

1 pepper

1 tomato

2 cups spinach

Procedure:

Juice the ingredients. Pour in a glass.

Chapter 5: Juicing Recipes For Boosting Metabolism

26. Tomato Basil Juice

Ingredients:

3 ripe tomatoes

8 basil leaves

1 apple

Procedure:

Chop the ingredients then process in a juicer.

27. Warm Apricot

Ingredients:

½ cup apricots

1 tsp honey

1 inch ginger

¾ cup milk

Procedure:

Juice the apricot and ginger. Stir in the honey and milk.

28. Tropical Booster

Ingredients:

1 mango

½ cup coconut milk

½ cup pineapple

Procedure:

Juice the fruits then add the milk.

29. Melon Berry Juice

Ingredients:

1 cup strawberries

1 ½ cups watermelon

¼ cup cantaloupe

Procedure:

Place in a juicer then process.

30.   Asparagus Delight

Ingredients:

3 carrots

4 spear asparagus

2 apples

1 celery stalk

Procedure:

Juice the ingredients then serve.

31.   Mexican Juice

Ingredients:

1 cup cilantro

Juice of ½ lime

2 medium apples

2 cucumbers

1 sweet pepper

Procedure:

Juice the ingredients. Add ice if desired.

32. Antioxidant Recipe

Ingredients:

1 pepper

2 carrots

Half cucumber

2 tomatoes

3 celery stalks

Procedure:

Place all the ingredients in a juicer.

33. Salad Juice

Ingredients:

5 lettuce leaf

3 tomatoes

1 onion

Half cucumber

1 sweet pepper

Procedure:

Juice the ingredients then serve.

34. Rainbow Blitz

Ingredients:

1 apple

1 cucumber

Juice from 1 lemon

2 cups spinach

1 pear

1 inch ginger, grated

Procedure:

Juice the ingredients. Stir then serve.

35. Tangerine juice

Ingredients:

1 tangerine

1 apple

Juice of 1 lemon

3 celery stalks

Procedure:

Juice the ingredients.

36. Apple Kale Juice

Ingredients:

1 tbsp lemon juice

3 apples

2 kale leaves

Procedure:

Juice the ingredients.

37. Spring cooler

Ingredients:

1 apple

1 cup mint

1 cucumber

Procedure:

Juice the ingredients.

38. Pineapple Jalapeno Juice

Ingredients:

1 cucumber

2 cups pineapple

5 kale leaves

1 jalapeno

Procedure:

Juice the ingredients.

39. Blackberry Kiwi Juice

Ingredients:

1 cup blackberry

1 pear

1 kiwi fruit

30 peppermint leaves

½ cup pineapple

Procedure:

Juice the ingredients

40. Broccoli Juice

Ingredients:

3 cups broccoli

4 apples

Procedure:

Juice the ingredients.

41. Celery Tomato Juice

Ingredients:

5 celery stalks

3 tomatoes

1 cucumber

Procedure:

Juice the ingredients.

42.Carrot Cabbage Delight

Ingredients:

Half cabbage head

3 carrots

Procedure:

Juice the ingredients.

43.Grape Spinach Juice

Ingredients:

2 cups grapes

2 cups spinach

1 avocado

1 tbsp honey

Procedure:

Juice the ingredients.

44.Licorice Love

Ingredients:

30 peppermint leaves

Half fennel bulb

2 apples

Procedure:

Juice the ingredients.

45. Bell Pepper Juice

Ingredients:

3 bell peppers

2 carrots

2 apples

Procedure:

Juice the ingredients

46. Almond Apple

Ingredients:

3 apples

½ cup almonds, crushed

Procedure:

Juice the apple. Add the almonds.

47. Blueberry Pineapple Juice

Ingredients:

2 cups blueberry

1 cup pineapple

1 cup spinach

Procedure:

Juice the ingredients.

48. Swiss Chard Juice

Ingredients:

5 Swiss chard leaves

1 apple

1 banana

Procedure:

Juice the ingredients.

Chapter 6: Detox Juice Recipes

49.Cilantro Detox

Ingredients:

10 cilantro sprigs

1 cup spinach

Procedure:

Combine in a juicer.

50.Strawberry Detox

Ingredients:

¾ cup strawberries

1 ½ cups kale

½ cup cucumber

1 banana

Procedure:

Juice the ingredients then pour in a glass.

51.   Blueberry Monster

Ingredients:

1 banana

½ cup blueberries

¼ cup mango

1 cup spinach

Procedure:

Juice the ingredients then pour in a glass.

52. Sweet cucumber
Ingredients:

2 handful of spinach

1 cucumber

2 small apples

Procedure:

Juice the ingredients.

53. Heart Beet
Ingredients:

1 apple

3 carrots

1 orange

1 beet root

Procedure:

Process the ingredients in a juicer.

54. Beet Spinach Juice

Ingredients:

1 cup spinach

1 beet root

1 apple

2 celery stalks

1 carrot

Procedure:

Place the ingredients in a juicer. Stir and serve.

55. Apple Beet Juice

Ingredients:

2 medium apples

2 carrots

Half cucumber

3 carrots

Procedure:

Juice the ingredients then pour in a glass

56. Cabbage Spinach Juice

Ingredients:

2 cups spinach 2 cabbage lead

½ cup pineapple

Lemon juice

Procedure:

Process the ingredients and stir.

57. Hang Under Juice

Ingredients:

2 celery stalks

2 cups spinach

1 tspspirulina

1 beet root

Procedure:

Process the ingredients in a juicer.

58. Morning Juice

Ingredients:

2 oranges

1 beet root

½ cup pineapple

Procedure:

Juice the ingredients.

59. Red Tangy Spice

Ingredients:

1 pepper

2 cups spinach

1 beet root

5 carrots

1 inch ginger

Procedure:

Process the ingredients in a juicer.

60. Liver Cleanse Juice

Ingredients:

1 inch ginger root

2 carrots

1 celery stalk

1 apple

1 beet green

Procedure:

Process it in a juicer.

61.   Beet retreat

Ingredients:

3 apples

2 beet roots

2 tbsp honey

Procedure:

Juice the apples and beet. Sweeten with honey.

62.Golden Spice Juice

Ingredients:

1 apple

1 inch ginger root

1 tsp pumpkin spice

Juice of half lemon

1 beet root

Procedure:

Process the ingredients in a juicer.

63.Hangover shot

Ingredients:

1 bitter melon

Half grapefruit

Juice of 1 lemon

Procedure:

Juice the fruits. Add the lemon juice and stir.

64.ABCD juice

Ingredients:

2 apples

1 beet

3 carrots

Procedure:

Juice the ingredients then serve.

65. Lemon Cleanse

Ingredients:

1 apple

1 inch ginger

3 carrots

Juice of 1 lemon

Procedure:

Process the ingredients then stir.

66. Parsley & Beets

Ingredients:

1 apple

2 celery stalks

1 beet root

1 cup parsley

3 carrots

Procedure:

Process the ingredients in a juicer.

67. Golden Beet Root Juice

Ingredients:

1 golden beet root

Half cucumber

1 pear

4 celery stalks

Procedure:

Process the ingredients in a juicer.

68.   Splendid Spinach

Ingredients:

2 apples

1 cup spinach

1 cup parsley

Procedure:

Place ingredients in a juicer then process

69.Strawberry Mint Juice

Ingredients:

12 peppermint leaves

2 cups strawberries

2 tbsp honey

2 tbsp lemon juice

Procedure:

Juice the fruits then add the honey.

Chapter 7: Juicing Recipes For Increasing Energy

70. Power up punch

Ingredients:

1/3 pineapple

2 lime

2 apples

1 cup spinach

Procedure:

Process the ingredients except for the lime. Squeeze the lime juice and add to the mixture.

71.   Afternoon pick-me-up

Ingredients:

2 apples

2 nectarines

2 kiwi fruits

½ cup pineapple

Procedure:

Remove stone from the nectarine. Process the ingredients and pour in a glass.

72. Mood Boosting Green Juice

Ingredients:

1 banana

1 tsp flaxseed

2 handful spinach

1 cup blueberries

1 cup organic milk

2 tbsp Greek yogurt

Procedure:

Combine banana, blueberries and spinach in a juicer. Add the remaining ingredients then stir.

73. Stress Relief Juice

Ingredients:

4 broccoli stalks

2 carrots

2 cups spinach

Procedure:

Juice and pour in a glass.

74. Turnip Fennel Juice

Ingredients:

3 carrots

1 apple

Half turnip

¼ fennel bulb

Procedure:

Wash and juice the ingredients.

75. Eggplant Carrot Juice

Ingredients:

1 celery stalk

2 apples

3 carrots

1 eggplant

Procedure:

Process the ingredients in the juicer.

76. Parsnip Carrot Juice

Ingredients:

1 apple

1 celery stalk

3 parsnips

3 carrots

Procedure:

Place the ingredients in a juicer and process.

77.   Decluttering Juice

Ingredients:

¼ cabbage head

½ inch ginger root

2 apples

4 cups spinach

Juice of half lemon

Procedure:

Juice all of the ingredients then stir.

78. Invigorating Juice

Ingredients:

1 lime

1 cup spinach

1 apple

1 cucumber

½ inch ginger

Half lemon

Procedure:

Juice the ingredients then serve.

79. Holiday lemonade

Ingredients:

½ cup cranberries

1 large orange

1 cup spinach

Juice of half lemon

Procedure:

Juice the ingredients.

80.   Peach medley

Ingredients:

2 apples

Half lemon

3 peaches

1 orange

Procedure:

Process the ingredients in a juicer.

81. Peachy Keen

Ingredients:

5 peaches

5 carrots

2 tbsp basil

Procedure:

Juice the ingredients then serve.

82.Purple Power

Ingredients:

¼ cabbage head

15 grapes

1 tbsp apple cider vinegar

1 apple

3 celery stalks

Procedure:

Juice the ingredients then serve.

83.Beginner Green

Ingredients:

5 cups spinach

2 bananas

1 orange

½ tsp lemon juice

Procedure:

Juice the ingredients then serve.

84.   Blood of Dragon

Ingredients:

4 red cabbage leaves

2 pears

1 tsp lemon juice

Procedure:

Process the ingredients in a juicer.

85. Lemon Ginger Zinger

Ingredients:

2 bananas

Half inch ginger root

2 carrots

3 tbsp lemon juice

Procedure:

Process the ingredients in a juicer.

86.   Mango Citrus Juice

Ingredients:

1 apple

1 mango

1 tbsp lemon juice

1 orange

Procedure:

Juice the fruits then add the lemon juice.

87. Pomegranate Juice

Ingredients:

1 cup pomegranate

1 banana

1 orange

Procedure:

Juice the fruits.

88. Orange Crush

Ingredients:

2 oranges

½ cup pineapple

1 peach

Procedure:

Juice the ingredients.

89. Peppermint Booster

Ingredients:

2 apples

10 peppermint leaves

1 inch ginger root

1 fennel bulb

Procedure:

Process the ingredients in a juicer

90. **Fruity Juice**
Ingredients:

2 apples

4 kiwis

2 oranges

1 cup pineapple

2 tbsp lemon juice

Procedure:

Process the ingredients in a juicer.

91. **Adios Coffee**
Ingredients:

1 apple

8 oz green tea

1 tsp honey

1 orange

4 carrots

1 tsp lemon juice

Procedure:

Make a cup of green tea. Juice the remaining ingredients then add to the green tea.

92.Blueberry Pomegranate

Ingredients:

1 cup blueberry

1 cup pomegranate

1 tbsp lemon juice

Procedure:

Juice the fruits then and the lemon juice.

Chapter 8: Healthy Juicing Recipes

93.Heavenly Chocolate Juice

Ingredients:

1 banana

1 cup sprig

1 mango

2 tbsp cocoa powder

½ cup raspberries

Procedure:

Process the ingredients in a juicer.

94.Pineapple-Kale- Cucumber Combo

Ingredients:

½ cup pineapple

1 apple

4 kale leaves

1 small cucumber

Procedure:

Chop ingredients then juice.

95.Pineapple Mint Juice

Ingredients:

4 kale leaves

1 cup pineapple

2 apples

2 cups spinach

Procedure:

Wash and juice the ingredients.

96.Celery Cucumber Juice

Ingredients:

½ cup cucumber

2 celery stalk

3 Swiss chard

2 kale leaves

1 banana

Procedure:

Juice the ingredients and add ice if desired.

97. Chia Kale Juice

Ingredients:

1 tspmaca

1 tsp chia seeds

8 oz hemp milk

4 kale leaves

1 banana

Procedure:

Process the banana and kale in a juicer. Add the remaining ingredients after.

98. Coconut Pomegranate Juice

Ingredients:

8 oz coconut water

1 tsp chia seeds

Half pomegranate

½ avocado

½ apple

Procedure:

Juice the ingredients then pour in a glass.

99.Banana Maca Juice

Ingredients:

8 oz hemp milk

2 tsp coconut flakes

1 banana

1 tspmaca powder

Procedure:

Juice the banana. Stir in the remaining ingredients.

100.   Avocado Juice

Ingredients:

Half avocado

1 pear

4 handful spinach

Procedure:

Place ingredients in a juicer then process.

101.   Goji Juice

Ingredients:

½ cup goji berries

1 banana

4 oz chilled green tea

Procedure:

Juice the fruits. Add the tea then stir.

102. Apple Cinnamon

Ingredients:

3 apples

2 tsp cinnamon

1 tsp chia seeds

1 banana

Procedure:

Juice the fruits then stir in the seed and cinnamon.

103. Sweet Potato Juice

Ingredients:

8 oz almond milk

½ cup cooked sweet potato

1 tsp coconut oil

1 banana

Procedure:

Juice the banana and cooked potato. Add the remaining ingredients.

104. Parsley juice

Ingredients:

1 cup parsley

½ cup pineapple

Lemon juice

Procedure:

Combine ingredients in a juicer.

105. Refreshing Cucumber Juice

Ingredients:

4 inch cucumber

¼ cup mint

Procedure:

Juice the ingredients and pour in a glass.

106. Cherry Green Juice

Ingredients:

1 cup cherries

1 cup milk

1 cup kale leaves

Procedure:

Combine the cherries and kale in a juicer. Stir in the milk.

107.   Pineapple Ginger Juice
Ingredients:

½ cup banana

1 cup pineapple

1 cup spinach

Juice of half lime

Procedure:

Pour the lime juice in the glass first. Juice the ingredients then add to glass.

108.   Orange Green Juice
Ingredients:

1 radish

1 green leaf

1 orange

1 tbsp chia seeds

Procedure:

Juice the ingredients.

109. Classic Kale

Ingredients:

3 apples

1 lemon

1 tbsp honey

5 kale stalks

Procedure:

Juice the apple and kale. Squeeze the lemon then add the honey.

110. Arthritis Soother

Ingredients:

1 apple

1 broccoli stalk

1 tbsp olive oil

3 large carrots

1 cup parsley

4 asparagus

Procedure:

Juice the ingredients then serve.

111. Breast Cancer Awareness Juice

Ingredients:

Juice of half lemon

1 large watermelon

1 large tomato

Procedure:

Juice the ingredients.

Chapter 9: Foods To Avoid

As a general rule, you should only juice foods that you would consume whole. However, there are some foods that you should avoid when it comes to juicing.

Citrus rinds

Citrus peels from oranges and grapefruit contain oil that can be difficult to digest for the stomach. It is highly recommended that you squeeze the juice from the citrus fruit manually then add it to the remaining ingredients. Lemon and lime is exempted from this since they are safe to be juiced whole.

Carrot greens

Cut the top part of the carrots since it is toxic to the body.

Papaya and pineapple peels

The peel of papaya is not edible. Pineapple peel can damage the juicer and can make it difficult to clean after.

Chapter 10: Tips And Tricks For Best Tasting Juices

Here are some tips and tricks to make delicious juices:

- Add herbs

Opt for herbs and spices instead of adding artificial ingredients in your juice. Herbs also have great therapeutic and medicinal benefit.

- Add citrus

Citrus fruits are rich in Vitamin C which can boost your immune system. It can also act as a natural preservative for your juice.

- Chop it first

Cutting the fruits and vegetable makes it easier to fit in the juicer. It also helps in breaking down the fruits and vegetables.

- Choose glass containers

Chemicals in plastic containers mix with the juice and can contaminate the juice. Opt to use glass bottles to keep you juice fresh.

- Do not overstuff the juicer

Overstuffing the juicer can put too much pressure on the machine. You can divide the ingredients into several batches and juice it separately.

Conclusion

Thank you again for purchasing the book juicing!

I am extremely excited to pass this information along to you, and I am so happy that you now have read and can hopefully implement these strategies going forward.

I hope this book was able to help you understand the benefits of fresh juice and how to make your own.

The next step is to get started using this information and to hopefully live a healthy life!

Please don't be someone who just reads this information and doesn't apply it, the strategies in this book will only benefit you if you use them!

If you know of anyone else that could benefit from the information presented here please inform them of this book.

Finally, if you enjoyed this book and feel it has added value to your life in any way, please take the time to share your thoughts and post a review on Amazon. It'd be greatly appreciated!

Thank you and good luck!

Preview Of:

50 Green Smoothie Diet Recipes!

<u>Green Smoothie Diet</u>

The Ultimate 5-Day Detox Dieting Guide To Improve Health, Boost Energy, Lose Weight, Kick Cravings, And Rejuvenate With Essential Smoothies!

.

Introduction

I want to thank you and congratulate you for purchasing the book, *"50 Green Smoothie Diet Recipes! - The Ultimate 5 Day Detox Dieting Guide to Improve Health, Boost Energy, Lose Weight, Kick Cravings, And Rejuvenate With Essential Smoothies!"*.

This "Green Smoothie Diet" book contains proven steps and strategies on how to heal your body, fight diseases, eliminate existing medical conditions, enhance your immunity, lose weight, regain your energy, improve your mood, jump start your metabolism, get rid of your cravings, fight the signs of aging, and achieve overall health and wellness by going on the Green Smoothie Diet.

You will learn how to do all these in just five days. Each day, you will focus on a specific benefit of the Green Smoothie Diet and learn how to make green smoothie recipes specifically formulated with that day's health focus in mind. At the end of five days, you will have detoxified your body, shed some pounds, gave your energy level a boost, and felt the immediate beneficial effects of super healing foods to your health and wellbeing.

This comprehensive guide contains tips and tricks on the proper preparation, consumption and storage of green smoothies. It also shows you how to make your smoothies extra scrumptious, how to get the optimum amount of nutrients from your smoothies, and how to make them in less time. Best of all, this book offers you 50 delicious and nutritious green smoothies to get you started on your diet! Excited? Flip the page and start now!

Thanks again for purchasing this book, I hope you enjoy it!

Chapter 1: What Is The Green Smoothie Diet?

Green smoothies have gone well past just being a diet trend. Today, many people know about their health benefits and are regular green smoothie drinkers. They aren't hard to find anymore either, as many cafes, restaurants, and juice bars now offer various green smoothie concoctions. Nutritionists and dieticians have acknowledged the beneficial effects of green smoothies, and there are thousands of articles on the Internet touting the healing powers of these amazing drinks.

Green Smoothies vs. "Green Smoothies"

However, before we discuss the Green Smoothie Diet, let's get one thing straight: overpriced, artificially sweetened drinks disguised as "green smoothies" are not the same as *real*, homemade, 100% natural green smoothies. The real deal does not contain artificial sweeteners, refined sugar, food coloring, ice cream and juice concentrates. Real, honest-to-goodness, health-boosting green smoothies are made with only the freshest, preferably organic vegetables and fruits blended together with well-chosen all-natural superfoods such as Spirulina and chia seeds. Unlike store-bought smoothies, there is no place in a real green smoothie for high fructose corn syrup or food dyes.

The Green Smoothie Diet

The challenge behind the Green Smoothie Diet is to drink at least one green smoothie a day. The reason behind it is that regular consumption of green smoothies helps you lose weight, makes you feel more energetic, improves your immunity, gives you a youthful glow, treats or reduces the symptoms of existing health issues, cleanses your body and just gives you an overall feeling of good health from the inside out.

Considerations

Green smoothies are great meal replacements, but replacing *all* your meals with smoothies is not recommended. These drinks, though nutrient-dense, do not have enough calories in them to replace your every meal. Anything that has fewer than 300 calories is not a fit meal. For best results, replace your breakfast and one other light meal (e.g. your afternoon snack) with a green smoothie. Any more than that and you are starving yourself.

Thanks For Previewing My Exciting Book Entitled:

"Green Smoothie Diet: 50 Green Smoothie Diet Recipes! The Ultimate 5-Day Detox Dieting Guide To Improve Health, Boost Energy, Lose Weight, Kick Cravings, And Rejuvenate With Essential Smoothies!"

To purchase this book, simply go to the Amazon Kindle store and simply search:

 "GREEN SMOOTHIE DIET"

Then just scroll down until you see my book. You will know it is mine because you will see my name "Chris Smith" underneath the title.

Alternatively, you can visit my author page on Amazon to see this book and other work I have done. Thanks so much, and please don't forget your free bonuses

DON'T LEAVE YET! - CHECK OUT YOUR FREE BONUSES BELOW!

Free Bonus Offer: Get Free Access To The www.LiveFitVIP.com VIP Newsletter!

Once you enter your email address you will immediately get free access to this awesome newsletter!

But wait, right now if you join now for free you will also get free access to the "The 7 Keys To Body Transformation" free EBook!

To claim both your FREE VIP NEWSLETTER MEMBERSHIP and your FREE BONUS EBook on THE 7 KEYS TO BODY TRANSFORMATION!

Just Go To:

www.liveFitVIP.com